HEALTHY LIVING

EFFECTIVE FOODS TO HELP YOU LOSE WEIGHT

VICTOR AJAYI

List of chapters

CHAPTER 1

Fat Burning Basics

In the event that you're overweight, you are not a terrible individual. You're just overweight. However, it's essential to lose the additional pounds so you'll look great, feel better and foster a deep satisfaction and confidence. Whenever you've lost the fat, you'll have to keep up with your weight.

In this booklet, you'll find how to shed 10 pounds per month - a decent, safe loss of around two or more than two pounds every week - effortlessly. You'll feel fulfilled and more lively than in the past without feeling denied.

Most Americans pack on those additional pounds by eating some unacceptable things. Changing these unfortunate dietary patterns is the way to long haul achievement. Information - alongside the right food - is the key.

At the point when people lived in caves, they knew nothing about protecting and putting away food. They invested all their waking investment hunting and assembling food. At the point when they had it, they ate it down quick. Rather than putting away food in storage rooms or pantries, they put away energy in their bodies as fat to consume during periods when nothing remained to be eaten.

Every year, it was totally indispensable for them to put on a decent layer of fat during the warm run and late spring months. That was the main way they could ensure their endurance during the lean and mean cold weather months.

Also, since ladies bore the youthful, they required more energy to support themselves and their infants, and that implied they were normally heavier.

Despite the fact that we presently not live in caves, we have acquired and kept up with this fundamental system for fat capacity from our hunting and assembling progenitors.

Every single one of us is brought into the world with a specific number of fat cells. The number of these fat cells you have relies upon hereditary qualities. In the event that you have a great deal of fat cells, perhaps your predecessors were the greatest individuals in the clan, which was something to be thankful for in light of the fact that they had the best possibilities of endurance.

You can never dispose of fat cells, yet - tragically - you can add to them. Contingent on what you eat, your body will make new far cells. Furthermore, similar to those you were brought into the world with, they never disappear.

That doesn't mean you're ill-fated to be fat once you put on additional pounds. Contracting fat cells is conceivable. That happens when you shed pounds. You consume the fat put away in those huge cells. Consider them inflatables. Consuming off the fat inside them has the save impact as letting the air out of an inflatable.

A decent get-healthy plan requires a specific measure of admission limitation - the utilization of less calories. You consume off the fat by eating less fat and turning out to be more dynamic.

To ensure a long period of weight-control a good outcome, you need to change the kind of food sources you eat, so you ingest less fat regardless get the nutrients, minerals, minor components, protein, fat and sugars your body needs to flourish.

Very low-calorie diets might assist you with shedding pounds rapidly, however they'll prompt disappointment over the long haul.

That is on the grounds that people are hereditarily safeguarded against starvation. During food deficiencies, our bodies delayed down our digestion systems and consume less energy so we can remain alive.

A piece of our cerebrum called the nerve center keeps us on an even weight keep by making a "set point." That's the weight where we feel good. The nerve center decides this point in light of the degree of utilization it's utilized to. It looks to keep our weight steady, regardless of whether that point is over what it ought to be.

At the point when we radically cut back our food consumption, the mind thinks the body is starving, and with an end goal to save life, it eases back the digestion. Before long the pounds quit falling off. Therefore, we become eager and awkward and afterward eat more. And afterward the eating routine falls flat.

How might you make up for this metabolic lull? The response is that you need to change the wholesome sythesis of the food sources you eat. You should eliminate all out calories - that is totally essential to weight reduction. More significant, notwithstanding, is diminishing the level of all out calories you are getting from fat.

That is the way you'll keep away from starvation alarm in your framework. Simultaneously, you diminish how much fat in your food, supplanting it with protected, low calorie, supplement rich plant food varieties. This will persuade your mind that your body is getting all the nourishment it needs.

As a matter of fact, you'll have the option to eat more food and feel more fulfilled while devouring less calories and fats.

Plant food varieties separate gradually in your stomach, encouraging you longer, and they are plentiful in nutrients, minerals, minor components, sugars and protein for energy and muscle-building. This permits your body to consume off its abundance put away fat.

CHAPTER 2

Every last one of the accompanying food varieties is clinically demonstrated to advance weight reduction. These food sources go a stage past essentially adding no fat to your framework - they have extraordinary properties that add hurdle to your framework and assist your body with dissolving away unfortunate pounds. These mind boggling food varieties can stifle your craving for low quality food and keep your body chugging along as expected with clean fuel and proficient energy.

You can remember these food sources for any reasonable weight reduction plan. They give your body the extra metabolic dismiss that it needs to rapidly shave from weight.

A reasonable weight reduction plan requires no less that 1,200 calories each day. In any case, Dr. Charles Klein suggests consuming more that that, on the off chance that you can trust it - 1,500 to 1,800 calories each day. He says you will in any case get in shape really at that admission level without jeopardizing your wellbeing.

Hunger is fulfilled all the more totally by filling the stomach. Ounce for ounce, the food sources recorded underneath achieve that better than any others. Simultaneously, they're wealthy in supplements and have extraordinary fat-softening abilities.

Apples

These wonders of nature merit their standing for fending the specialist off when you eat one per day. Also, presently, it appears, they can assist you with liquefying the fat away, as well.

They, first of all, raise your blood glucose (sugar) levels in a protected, delicate way and keep them up longer than most food sources. The down to earth impact of this is to leave you feeling fulfilled longer, say scientists.

Also, they're one of the most extravagant wellsprings of solvent fiber in the grocery store. This kind of fiber forestalls food cravings by making preparations for risky swings or drops in your glucose level, says Dr. James Anderson of the University of Kentucky's School of Medicine.

A typical size apple gives just 81 calories and has no sodium, soaked fat or cholesterol. You'll likewise get the additional medical advantages of bringing down the degree of cholesterol currently in your blood along with bringing down your circulatory strain.

Entire Grain Bread

You shouldn't even need to fear bread. It's the spread, margarine or cream cheddar you put on it that is swelling, not the actual bread. We'll express this as frequently on a case by case basis - fat is swelling. On the off chance that you don't really accept that that, contemplate this - a gram of sugar has four calories, a gram of protein four, and a gram of fat nine. So which of these is truly swelling?

Bread, a characteristic wellspring of fiber and complex sugars, is acceptable as far as slimming down. Norwegian researcher Dr. Bjarne Jacobsen found that individuals who eat under two cuts of bread everyday weigh around 11 pounds more that the people who eat a ton of bread.

Learns at Michigan State University show a few breads really lessen the hunger. Specialists contrasted white bread with dim, high-fiber bread and found that understudies who ate 12 cuts per day of the dim, high-fiber bread felt less craving consistently and shed five pounds in two months. Other people who ate white bread were hungrier, ate additional swelling food varieties and lost no weight during this time.

So the key is eating dull, rich, high-fiber breads like pumpernickel, entire wheat, blended grain, cereal and others. The typical cut of entire grain bread contains simply 60 to 70 calories, is wealthy in complex starches - the best, steadiest fuel you can give your body - and conveys astounding measure of protein.

Espresso

Simple does it is the secret phrase here. We've all found out about possible risks of caffeine - including tension and a sleeping disorder - so balance is the key.

The caffeine in espresso can accelerate the digestion. In wholesome circles, it's known as a metabolic enhancer, as per Dr. Judith Stern of the University of California at Davis.

This checks out, since caffeine is an energizer. Concentrates on show it can assist you with consuming a greater number of calories than ordinary, maybe up to 10 percent more. For the wellbeing of security, restricting your admission to a solitary cup in the first part of the day and one PM is ideal. Add just skim milk to tit and take a stab at managing without sugar - many individuals figure out how to cherish it that way.

Grapefruit

There's valid justification for this customary eating regimen food to be a normal piece of your eating routine. It assists disintegrate with fatting and cholesterol, as indicated by Dr. James Cerd of the University of Florida. A typical estimated grapefruit has 74 calories, conveys an astounding 15 grams of gelatin (the extraordinary fiber connected to bringing down cholesterol and fat), is high in L-ascorbic acid and potassium and is liberated from fat and sodium.

It's wealthy in normal galacturonic corrosive, which adds to its power as a fat and cholesterol warrior. The extra advantage here is help with the fight against atherosclerosis (solidifying of the conduits) and the improvement of coronary illness. Have a go at sprinkling it with cinnamon as opposed to sugar to remove a portion of the tart taste.

Mustard

Try the hot, spicy kind you find in Asian import stores, stores and exotic foods. Dr. Jaya Henry of Oxford Polytechnic Institute in England, found that how much hot mustard typically called for in Mexican, Indian and Asian recipes, around one teaspoon, briefly accelerates the digestion, similarly as.

"Be that as it may, mustard is normal and absolutely protected," Henry says. "It very well may be utilized consistently, and it truly works. I was stunned to find it can accelerate the digestion by as much as 20 to 25 percent for a few hours." This can bring about the body consuming an extra 45 calories for each 700 consumed, Dr. Henry says.

Peppers

Peppers

Hot, fiery bean stew peppers fall into a similar classification as hot mustard, Henry says. He concentrated on them under similar conditions as the mustard and they worked comparably well. A simple three grams of bean stew peppers were added to a feast comprising of 766 complete calories. The peppers' digestion raising properties worked like a

 engage, prompting what Henry calls an eating regimen incited thermic impact. It doesn't produce a lot to make the results. Most salsa recipes call for four to eight chilies - that is not much.

Peppers are incredibly plentiful in nutrients An and C, bountiful in calcium, phosphorus, iron and magnesium, high in fiber, liberated from fat, low in sodium and have only 24 calories for every cup.

Potatoes

We must youngster, isn't that so? Wrong. Potatoes have fostered something very similar "swelling" rap as bread, and it's unreasonable. Dr. John McDougal, overseer of the dietary medication facility at St. Helena Hospital in Deer Park,

California, says, "A magnificent food with which to accomplish quick weight reduction is the potato, at 0.6 calories per gram or around 85 calories for every potato." An extraordinary wellspring of fiber and potassium, they lower cholesterol and safeguard against strokes and coronary illness.

Planning and fixings are essential. Avoid margarine, milk and sharp cream, or you'll blow it. Select yogurt all things being equal.

Rice

A whole weight reduction plan, basic called the Rice Diet, was created by Dr. William Kempner at Duke University in Durham, North Carolina. The eating regimen, dating to the 1930's, makes rice the staple of your food consumption. Later on, you continuously blend in different foods grown from the ground.

It produces dazzling weight reduction and clinical outcomes. The eating routine has been displayed to opposite and fix kidney Illnesses and hypertension.

A cup of cooked rice (150 grams) contains around 178 calories - roughly 33% the quantity of calories tracked down in a comparable measure of meat or cheddar. What's more, recall, entire grain rice is vastly improved for you than white rice.

Soup is really great for you! Perhaps not the canned assortments from the store - however antiquated, custom made soup advances weight reduction. A concentrate by Dr. John Foreyt of Baylor College of Medicine in Houston, Texas, found that calorie counters who ate a bowl of soup before lunch and supper lost more weight than health food nuts who didn't. Truth be told, the more soup they ate, the more weight they lost. Also, soup eaters will generally keep the load off longer.

Normally, the kind of soup you eat has an effect. Cream soups or those made of hamburger or pork are not your smartest options. Yet, here's an incredible recipe:

Cut three enormous onions, three carrots, four stems of celery, one zucchini and one yellow squash. Place in a pot. Add three jars squashed tomatoes, two bundles low-sodium chicken bouillon, three jars water and one cup white wine (discretionary). Add tarragon, basil, oregano, thyme and garlic powder. Bubble, then, at that point, stew for 60 minutes. Serves six.

Spinach

Popeye truly understood what he was referring to, as per Dr. Richard Shekelle, a disease transmission specialist at the University of Texas. Spinach can bring down cholesterol, fire up the digestion and consume with smoldering heat fat. Plentiful in iron, beta carotene and nutrients C and E, it supplies a large portion of the supplements you really want.

Tofu

You can't express sufficient about this wellbeing food from Asia. Likewise called soybean curd, it's fundamentally boring, so any zest or enhancing you add mixes with it pleasantly. A 2½ " square has 86 calories and nine grams of protein. (Specialists recommend an admission of around 40 grams each day.) Tofu contains calcium and iron, basically no sodium and no immersed fat. It makes your digestion run on high and even brings down cholesterol. With various assortments accessible, the firmer tofus are goof for pan-searing or adding to soups and sauces while the milder ones are really great for crushing, hacking and adding to servings of mixed greens.

CHAPTER 3

It would be ridiculous to figure you could effectively get more fit and appreciate what you're eating with a simple modest bunch of food sources, regardless of how flavorful, nutritious and fulfilling they might be. So we will add an additional program of fat-battling food varieties you can eat alongside the extraordinary food varieties referenced in the last area.

They'll loan various preferences and surfaces to each dinner and give a large number of nutrients, minerals, proteins and other crucial supplements. Normally, every one is high in fiber, low in fat and safe with regards to sodium content, as well.

Many have crunchiness and flavor we've come to want in nibble and snacking food varieties. In the event that you're like the majority of us, you might have a genuine low quality food eating propensity - a propensity you must change to thin down. A significant number of the food sources in this segment might be commendable substitutes.

This filling grain piles up well to rice and potatoes. It has 170 calories for every cooked cup, good degrees of protein and fiber and generally low fat. Roman warriors ate this grain routinely for strength and really grumbled when they needed to eat meat.

Learns at the University of Wisconsin show that grain really brings cholesterol by up down to 15 percent and has strong enemy of disease specialists. Israeli researchers say it fixes clogging better compared to intestinal medicines - and that can advance weight reduction, as well.

Use it as a substitute for rice in plates of mixed greens, pilaf or stuffing, or add to soups and stews. You can likewise blend it in with rice for a fascinating surface. Ground into flour, it makes fantastic breads and biscuits.

Beans are one of the most amazing wellsprings of plant protein. Peas, beans and chickpeas are on the whole known as vegetables. Most normal beans have 215 calories for every cooked cup (lima beans go up to 260). They have the most protein with the most un-fat of any food, and they're high in potassium yet low in sodium.

Plant protein is fragmented, and that implies that you want to add something to make it complete. Consolidate beans with an entire grain - rice, grain, wheat, corn - to give the amino acids important to shape a total protein. Then, at that point, you get a similar top-quality protein as in meat with simply a small part of the fat.

Learns at the University of Kentucky and in the Netherlands demonstrate the way that eating beans consistently can bring down cholesterol levels.

The most well-known grievance about beans is that they cause gas. This is the way to contain that issue, as per the U.S. Branch of Agriculture (USDA): Before cooking, flush the beans and eliminate unfamiliar particles, put in a pot and cover with bubbling water, drench for four hours or longer, eliminate any beans that float to the top, then, at that point, cook the beans in new water.

Berries

This is the ideal weight reduction food. Berries have normal fructose sugar that fulfills your yearning for desserts and enough fiber so you assimilate less calories that you eat. English analysts found that the high satisfied of insoluble fiber in organic products, vegetables and entire grains lessens the retention of calories from food sources enough to advance width misfortune without hampering nourishment.

Berries are an extraordinary wellspring of potassium that can help you in circulatory strain control. Blackberries have 74 calories for every cup, blueberries 81, raspberries 60 and strawberries 45. So utilize your creative mind and partake in your preferred berry.

Broccoli

Broccoli is America's number one vegetable, as indicated by a new survey. No big surprise. A cup of cooked broccoli has a simple 44 calories. It conveys a stunning healthful payload and is viewed as the main disease battling vegetable. It has no fat, heaps of fiber, malignant growth battling synthetic substances called indoles, carotene, multiple times the RDA of L-ascorbic acid and calcium.

While you're purchasing broccoli, focus on the variety. The minuscule florets ought to be rich green and free of yellowing. It would be ideal for stems to be firm.

Buckwheat

It's perfect for hotcakes, breads, oat, soups or alone as a grain dish generally called kasha. It has 155 calories for every cooked cup. Research at the All India Institute of Medical Sciences shows slims down including buckwheat lead to brilliant glucose guideline, protection from diabetes and brought down cholesterol levels. You cook buckwheat the same way you would rice or grain. Heat a few cups of water to the point of boiling, add the grain, cover the container, turn down the intensity and stew for 20 minutes or until the water is consumed.

Cabbage

This Eastern Europe staple is a genuine miracle food. There are just 33 calories in a cup of cooked destroyed cabbage, and it holds generally its healthful goodness regardless of how long you cook it. Eating cabbage crude (18 calories for every destroyed cup), cooked, as sauerkraut (27 calories for each depleted cup) or coleslaw (calories rely upon dressing) just once seven days is sufficient to safeguard against colon disease. What's more, it very well might be a life span upgrading food. Reviews in the United States, Greece and Japan show that individuals who eat a ton of it have the least colon malignant growth and the most minimal demise rates generally speaking.

Carrots

What rundown of wellbeing advancing, fat-battling food varieties could be finished without Bugs Bunny's #1? A medium-sized carrot conveys around 55 calories and is a healthful force to be reckoned with. The orange variety comes from beta carotene, a strong disease forestalling supplement (provitamin A).

Cleave and throw them with pasta, grind them into rice or add them to a sautéed food. Consolidate them with parsnips, oranges, raisins, lemon juice, chicken, potatoes, broccoli or sheep to make tasty dishes. Flavor them with tarragon, dill, cinnamon or nutmeg. Add finely cleaved carrots to soups and spaghetti sauce - they give a characteristic pleasantness without adding sugar.

Chicken

 White meat contains 245 calories for every four ounce serving and dim meat, 285. It's a phenomenal wellspring of protein, iron, niacin and zinc. Cleaned chicken is best, yet most specialists prescribe holding on until subsequent to cooking to eliminate it in light of the fact that the skin keeps the meat wet during cooking.

Corn

It's actually a grain - not a vegetable - and is another food that is gotten a bum rap. Individuals think it brings essentially nothing to the table healthfully and that simply isn't really. There are 178 calories in a cup of cooked parts. It contains great measures of iron, zinc and potassium, and University of Nebraska specialists say it conveys a top notch of protein, as well.

The Tarahumara Indians of Mexico eat corn, beans and practically nothing else. Virgil Brown, M.D., of Mount Sinai School of Medicine in New York, calls attention to that high blood cholesterol and cardiovascular coronary illness are practically nonexistent among them.

Curds

However long we're looking at shedding pounds and fat-battling food sources, we needed to make reference to curds.

Low-fat (2%) curds has 205 calories for each cup and is commendably low in fat, while giving decent measures of calcium and the B nutrient riboflavin. Season with flavors such a dill, or nursery new vegetable such a scallions and chives for additional zip.

To make it better, add raisins or one of the natural product spreads with no sugar added. You can likewise utilize curds in cooking, baking, fillings and plunges where you would somehow utilize acrid cream or cream cheddar.

Figs

Fiber-rich figs are low in calories at 37 for each medium (2.25" width) crude fig and 48 for every dried fig. A new report by the USDA showed that they add to a sensation of completion and forestall indulging. Subjects really griped of being approached to eat a lot of food when taken care of an eating regimen containing a larger number of figs than a comparative eating regimen with an indistinguishable number of calories.

Serve them with different foods grown from the ground. Or on the other hand poach them in natural product squeeze and serve them warm or cold. You can stuff them with gentle white cheddar or puree them to use as a filling for treats and low-calorie cakes.

Fish

The medical advantages of fish are more prominent than specialists envisioned - and they've generally thought of it as a wellbeing food.

The carbohydrate level in the normal four-ounce serving of a remote ocean fish runs from a low of 90 calories in abalone to a high of 236 in herring. Water-stuffed fish, for instance, has 154 calories. It's difficult to put on weight eating fish.

As far back as 1985, articles in the New England Journal of Medicine showed an unmistakable connection between eating fish routinely and lower paces of coronary illness. The explanation is that oils in fish slim the blood, decrease pulse and lower cholesterol.

 Dr. Joel Kremer, at Albany Medical College in New York, found that day to day enhancements of fish oil carried emotional help to the irritation and firm joints of rheumatoid joint pain.

Greens

We're talking collard, chicory, beet, kale, mustard, Swiss chard and turnip greens. They all have a place with a similar family as spinach, and that is one of the hotshots. Regardless of how enthusiastically you attempt, you can't stack a cup of plain cooked greens with anything else than 50 calories.

They're brimming with fiber, stacked with nutrients An and C, and liberated from fat. You can involve them in plates of mixed greens, soups, goulashes or any dish where you would typically utilize spinach.

Kiwi

This New Zealand local is a sweet treat at just 46 calories for each organic product. Chinese general wellbeing authorities acclaim the delectable organic product for its high L-ascorbic acid substance and potassium. It stores effectively in the fridge for as long as a month. A great many people like it stripped, however the fluffy skin is additionally consumable.

These individuals from the onion family seem to be monster scallions, and are just as stimulating and delightful as their better-known cousins. They come as near without calorie as it gets at a simple 32 calories for each cooked cup.

You can poach or sear divided leeks and afterward marinate them in vinaigrette or season with Romano cheddar, fine mustard or spices. They likewise make a decent soup.

Individuals think lettuce is healthfully useless, however nothing could be farther from reality. You can't avoid it with regards to your weight reduction plans, not at 10 calories for each cup of crude romaine. It gives a ton of filling mass for scarcely any calories. Also, it's brimming with L-ascorbic acid, as well. Go past chunk of ice lettuce with Boston, bibb and cos assortments or attempt watercress, arugula, radicchio, dandelion greens, purslane and even parsley to spice up your plates of mixed greens.

Presently, here's extraordinary taste and extraordinary sustenance in a low-calorie bundle! One cup of melon balls has 62 calories, on cup of casaba balls has 44 calories, one cup of honeydew balls has 62 calories and one cup of watermelon balls has 49 calories. They have probably the most elevated fiber content of any food and are heavenly. Toss in attractive amounts of nutrients An and C in addition to an incredible 547 mgs of potassium in that cup of melon, and you have a fat-consuming wellbeing food unparalleled.

Oats

A cup of oats or oat wheat has just 110 calories. What's more, oats assist you with getting in shape. Subjects in Dr. James Anderson's milestone 12-year learn at the University of Kentucky shed three pounds in two months essentially by adding 100 grams (3.5 ounces) of oat wheat to their everyday food admission and that's it. Simply don't expect oats alone to perform supernatural occurrences - you need to eat a decent eating routine for all out wellbeing.

Onions

Delightful, fragrant, modest and low in calories, onions merit a standard spot in your eating routine. One cup of slashed crude onions has just 60 calories, and one crude medium onion (2.15" distance across) has only 42.

They control cholesterol, flimsy the blood, safeguard against cholesterol and may have some worth in balancing

unfavorably susceptible responses. In particular, onions taste
great and they're really great for you.

Somewhat bubble, strip and prepare, seasoning with olive oil
and lemon juice. Or on the other hand sauté them in white
wine and basil, then spread over pizza. Or on the other hand
broil them in sherry and serve over glue.

Pasta

The Italians had it right from the start. A cup of cooked glue
(without a weighty sauce) has just 155 calories and fits the
depiction of an ideal starch-focused staple. Examination at
the American Institute of Baking shows pasta is plentiful in
six minerals, including manganese, iron, phosphorus, copper,
magnesium and zinc. Likewise make certain to consider
entire wheat pastas, which are significantly better.

Yams

You can make a dinner out of them and not stress over
acquiring a pound - and you sure won't leave the table
inclination hungry. Every yam has around 103 calories. Their
velvety orange tissue is one of the most mind-blowing
wellsprings of vitamin A you can consume.

You can prepare, steam or microwave them. Or on the other hand add them to goulashes, soups and numerous different dishes. Flavor with lemon juice or vegetable stock rather than spread.

Tomatoes

A medium tomato (2.5" measurement) has something like 25 calories. These nursery delights are low in fat and sodium, high in potassium and wealthy in fiber.

A review at Harvard Medical School observed that the possibilities passing on from malignant growth are most minimal among individuals who eat tomatoes (or strawberries) consistently.

Furthermore, don't ignore canned squashed, stripped, entire or stewed tomatoes. They make sauces, goulashes and soups taste perfect while holding their healthful goodness and low-calorie status. Indeed, even regular spaghetti sauce is a fat-consuming deal when served over pasta, so ponder bringing tomatoes into your eating regimen

Turkey

Express appreciation to those pioneers for beginning the superb custom of Thanksgiving turkey. Coincidentally this wellbeing food camouflaged as meat is great all year for weight control.

A four-ounce serving of simmered white meat turkey has 177 calories and dim meat has 211.

Unfortunately, numerous people are as yet ignorant about the adaptability and kind of ground turkey. Anything cheeseburger can do, ground turkey can do in some measure too, from ordinary burgers to spaghetti sauce to meat portion.

 Some ground turkey contains skin which marginally builds the fat substance. To keep it truly lean, settle on ground bosom meat. Yet, since this has no additional fat, you'll have to add filler to make burgers or meat portion keep intact.

Four ounces of ground turkey has around 170 calories and nine grams of fat - about what you'd track down in 2.5 teaspoons of spread or margarine. Unbelievably, a similar measure of ordinary ground meat (21% fat) has 298 calories and 23 grams of fat.

Purchasing turkey has become simple. It's presently not important to purchase an entire bird except if you have any desire to. Ground turkey is accessible new or frozen, as are individual pieces of the bird, including drumsticks, thighs, bosoms and cutlets.

The non-fat variety of plain yogurt has 120 calories for every cup and low-fat, 144. It conveys a great deal of protein and , like any dairy food, is wealthy in calcium and contains zinc and riboflavin.

Yogurt is helpful as a morning meal food - cut a banana into it and add your preferred cereal.

You can track down ways of involving it in different kinds of cooking, to - sauces, soups, plunges, garnishes, stuffings and spreads. Numerous kitchen device offices even sell a basic channel for making yogurt cheddar.

Yogurt can supplant weighty creams and entire milk in many dishes, saving scads of fat and calories.

You can substitute half or the higher fat fixings as a whole. Be imaginative. For instance, join yogurt, garlic powder, lemon squeeze, a hint of pepper and Worcestershire sauce and use it to top a prepared potato as opposed to heaping on fat-loaded sharp cream.

General stores and wellbeing food stores sell various yogurts, numerous with added products of the soil. To control calories and fat substance, purchase plain non-fat yogurt and add natural product yourself. Creamy fruit spread or natural product spreads with practically no additional sugar are a great method for transforming plain yogurt into a heavenly sweet treat.

www.ingramcontent.com/pod-product-compliance
Lightning Source LLC
Chambersburg PA
CBHW052136150726
48002CB00006B/2638